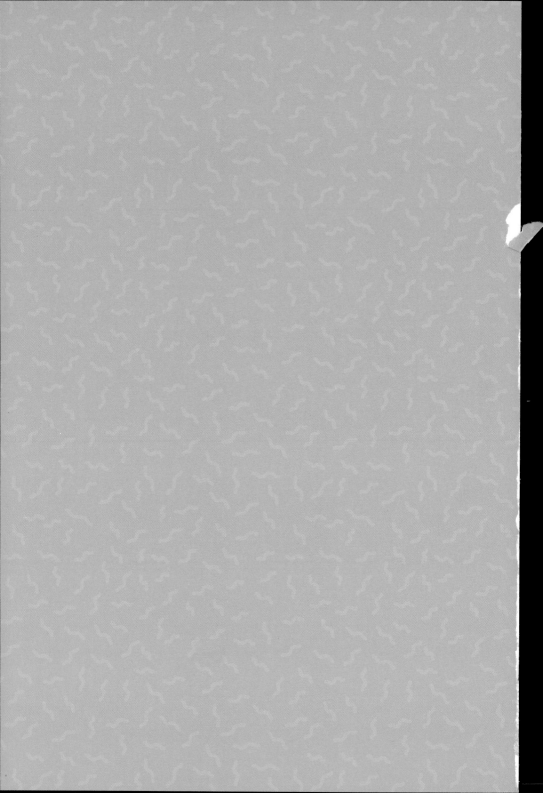

Baby on Board

9-Month Pregnancy Journal & Guide

FIVE MILE

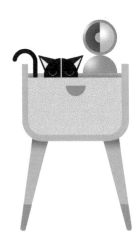

Made with love by the team at

FIVE MILE

Michelle, Rocco, Jacqui, Graham, Claire, Sarah, Bridget, Tillie, Kate & Victoria

Five Mile,
the publishing division
of Regency Media
www.fivemile.com.au

A catalogue record for this book is available from the National
Library of Australia

Printed in China 5 4 3 2 1

Baby on Board

9-Month Pregnancy Journal & Guide

FIVE MILE

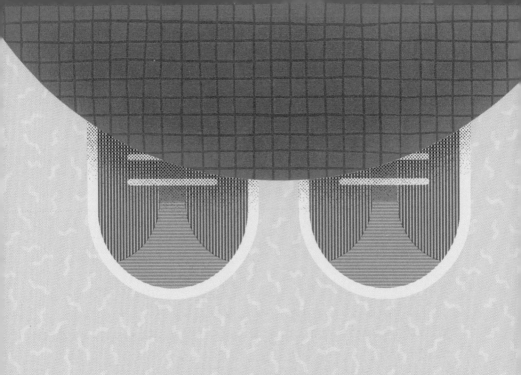
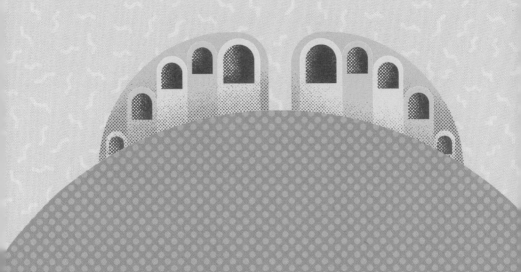

How to Use This Journal

Dear reader,

What you are holding is a journal that will accompany you for the next nine months. The first section will help see you through week after week of this wonderful journey, while the second will show you your monthly milestones.

There are no writing rules for you to follow in filling out these pages, but our advice is to be honest and not to be impersonal. Open your heart and let it shine in what you write—in the future, the child you are expecting can enjoy reading it, too.

Use the journal to reflect about yourself and your desires, about the future you want for your family and about the people who make you feel good. Enjoy the journey!

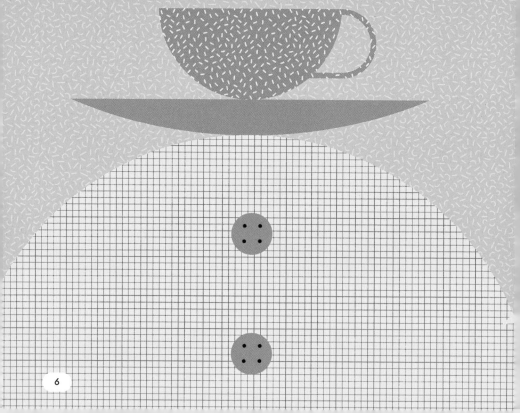

The Weeks

Pregnancy is a journey of transformation that, week by week, accompanies you toward childbirth. Live it to the fullest: write down everything you feel, everything you experience, all of your hopes. It makes no difference whether you have just found out you are pregnant or you are already well along in your pregnancy; use this section to record each stage so that you remember it in the future. There is also space devoted to medical appointments, ultrasound scans and shopping and to-do lists. Let's do this!

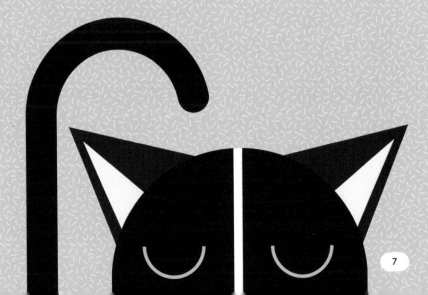

Strawberries at 3 a.m.?

Nutrition when you're pregnant!

All right! If there are no health implications, satisfy those surprise cravings for strawberries, chocolate, and pickles that surprise you at 3 a.m.! But let's dispel a myth right away: not satisfying your cravings does not lead to birthmarks on your baby. Cravings are not whims! During the nine months of pregnancy, your appetite and your relationship with food change dramatically.

Have you ever heard of toxoplasmosis?

Toxoplasmosis is a disease that can compromise foetal development. It is transmitted to humans through animals, especially cats (be careful cleaning the litter box) and food. How to avoid it? Wash fruits, vegetables, and fresh herbs to remove any traces of soil. Clean surfaces and kitchen utensils well after each use. Avoid eating raw meat and fish, cold cuts, raw milk and soft cheeses made from unpasteurised milk.

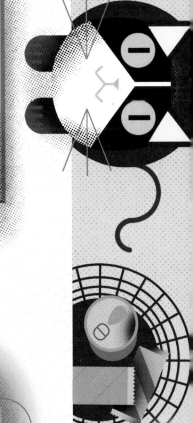
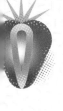

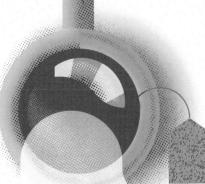

If you feel nauseated, try:

- eating small portions and often
- drinking a herbal tea with ginger
- thinking about food that appeals to you
- choosing light, fresh foods
- drinking slowly and regularly; and remember—it will go away soon!

Products to avoid:

- products with preservatives or palm oil
- phytosterol-rich products
- artificial sweeteners in soft drinks.
- Also beware of soy-based foods: no more than one a day! The phytoestrogens contained in them may interfere with your hormonal system.

First week
Date: ....

Shopping list:

1.
2.
3.
4.
5.

6.
7.
8.
9.
10.

Visits and things to do:

....
....
....
....
....
....
....
....
....

How you feel:

MONDAY

TUESDAY

WEDNESDAY

THURSDAY

FRIDAY

SATURDAY

SUNDAY

Your recipes for the week

....
....
....
....
....
....
....
....

....
....
....
....
....
....
....

....
....
....
....
....
....
....
....
....
....
....

....
....
....
....
....
....
....
....
....
....
....

Second week
Date: ....

Nutrition:

FOODS TO AVOID
IF YOU'RE
NAUSEATED:

FOODS THAT
MAKE YOUR
NAUSEA GO AWAY:

Your first symptoms:

Appointments:

....

MONDAY

....

TUESDAY

....

WEDNESDAY

....

THURSDAY

....

FRIDAY

....

SATURDAY

....

SUNDAY

How did you find out you were pregnant?

....

....

....

....

....

....

....

....

....

....

....

....

....

....

....

....

....

....

Third week

Date: ....

Shopping list:

1.

2.

3.

4.

5.

6.

7.

8.

9.

10.

What you like about being pregnant:

....
....
....
....
....
....
....
....
....

What you DON'T like about being pregnant:

....
....
....
....
....
....
....
....
....

A picture of you in your third week of pregnancy

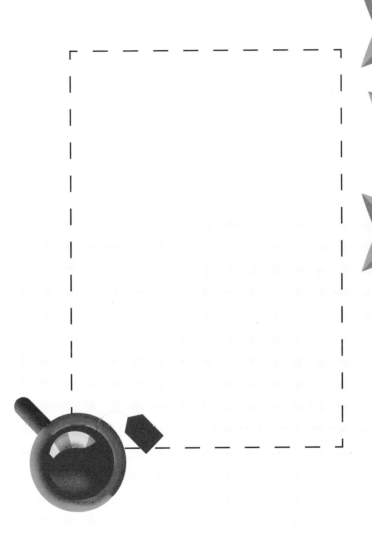

Fourth week
Date: ....

Changes and hopes:

....

....

....

....

How often are you drinking water?

MONDAY

TUESDAY

WEDNESDAY

THURSDAY

FRIDAY

SATURDAY

SUNDAY

How often are you walking?

MONDAY

TUESDAY

WEDNESDAY

THURSDAY

FRIDAY

SATURDAY

SUNDAY

Movies about pregnancy to watch

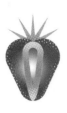

Hop! Hop! Get Moving!

Exercise during pregnancy!

If you are lazy, get moving, but if you are hyperactive, take it easy! Avoid violent or contact sports and focus on swimming, water aerobics, yoga, long walks, dance, or gentle gymnastics! Moderation is the key!

The exercise ball is your friend!

From your first trimester through labour, the exercise ball will become your best friend for relieving back tension, stretching, toning your abdominal muscles, and relaxing, all to the sound of "boing boing." Sit on the exercise ball like a chair; it will force you to maintain proper posture in your back. In a sitting position, swing your pelvis side to side while keeping your shoulders still.

From a seated position, rotate your hips clockwise and counterclockwise.

On your knees, bend over the ball while also supporting yourself with your arms.

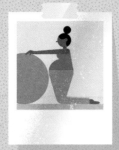

Why be active? It feels so good here on the couch!

There are at least five benefits to being active:
- it helps keep extra weight off and reduces the risk of gestational diabetes
- it lowers blood pressure
- it improves circulation
- it helps prevent back pain
- it improves your psychological well-being.

Lie down on the floor and rest your legs on the ball, then raise your upper body while keeping your hips resting on the floor.

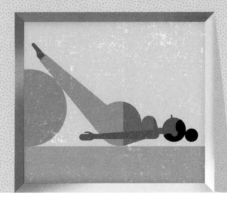

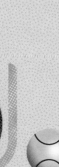

Sports to avoid:

Sports that carry a risk of falling or trauma and intense cardio activities: martial arts, combat sports, team sports, skiing, surfing, horseback riding, and aerobics.

Avoid high-altitude mountain sports and free diving during pregnancy — the lack of oxygen could harm the foetus.

Fifth week
Date: ....

Your favorite sports:

1. ....
2. ....
3. ....
4. ....
5. ....

6. ....
7. ....
8. ....
9. ....
10. ....

Your physical activities this week:

MONDAY

TUESDAY

WEDNESDAY

THURSDAY

FRIDAY

SATURDAY

SUNDAY

People who know you are pregnant:

....
....
....
....
....
....
....
....
....
....

Your recipes for the week

....
....
....
....
....
....
....
....
....
....
....
....
....
....
....
....
....
....
....
....

Sixth week

Date: ....

What physical activities can you do?

Activities OK:

1.

2.

3.

Activities NOT OK:

1.

2.

3.

Remember to:

....

....

....

....

....

....

....

....

....

....

Appointments:

....

....

....

....

....

....

....

....

....

....

Checklist for your second month of pregnancy

Seventh week

Date: ....

Shopping list:

....

....

....

....

....

....

....

....

....

....

**Correct nutrition
for physical activities:**

What NOT to eat:

....

....

....

....

....

....

....

....

1.

2.

3.

4.

5.

6.

7.

Attach a picture of yourself here

Eighth week
Date: ....

This week's physical activities:

....
....
....
....
....

How often are you drinking water?

MONDAY

TUESDAY

WEDNESDAY

THURSDAY

FRIDAY

SATURDAY

SUNDAY

How often are you walking?

MONDAY

TUESDAY

WEDNESDAY

THURSDAY

FRIDAY

SATURDAY

SUNDAY

Where do you like to go for a walk? List your favourite places

....
....
....
....
....
....

....
....
....
....
....
....

....
....
....
....
....
....

....
....
....
....
....
....

I'm Happy—No, Wait, I'm Sad!

Better known as mood swings in pregnancy!

Welcome to the roller coaster of pregnancy! Instead of holding on, learn to let go. When you are pregnant, particularly in your first and third trimesters, emotional "ups and downs" are completely normal.

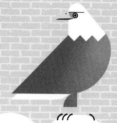

What can you do about these mood swings?

There is no way to counteract the side effects of hormones in pregnancy, so you will need to find some strategies for managing the many emotions you are experiencing.

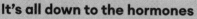

It's all down to the hormones

You may already know that hormones affect your mood. And since your body produces so many during pregnancy, it's easy to experience a wide range of emotions that can range from anger to enthusiasm, from anxiety to serenity, from extreme irritability to zen-like calm, from hatred to unconditional love for the whole world. Hormones may also make you feel more tired than usual, less focused and out of sorts.

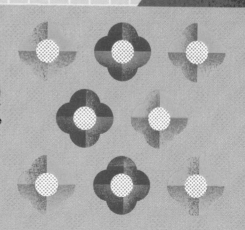

Talking about it helps

Instead of burying your negative feelings, try talking about them. Often, simply sharing them is enough to make them go away. Sometimes talking to a friend is not enough; if that is the case, make an appointment to talk to a psychologist.

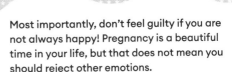

Most importantly, don't feel guilty if you are not always happy! Pregnancy is a beautiful time in your life, but that does not mean you should reject other emotions.

Here are some ideas:
- Try prenatal yoga, mindfulness practices or meditation: it only takes twenty minutes to regain the clarity you need to face the day.
- The best way to get help is to ask for help! If you feel restless, talk to your gynaecologist or midwife. They will know how to help you.

- Don't neglect your diet, which should always be balanced. Favour foods that can cheer you up, as some can be rich in magnesium, such as dark chocolate, bananas, wheat germ, legumes or rich in omega-3, such as eggs, chia seeds and fish.
- Rest, take time to engage in an activity that cheers you up without being too hard on yourself: even if it means giving up other daily activities.

Ninth week
Date: ....

How can you take care of yourself?

....
....
....
....
....
....

Visits and things to do:

How you feel:

MONDAY

....

TUESDAY

....

WEDNESDAY

....

THURSDAY

....

FRIDAY

....

SATURDAY

....

SUNDAY

....

Movies to watch

....
....
....
....
....
....
....
....
....
....
....
....
....
....
....
....
....
....

Tenth week

Date: ....

Little daily challenges:

1.

2.

3.

4.

5.

6.

7.

8.

Visits and things to do:

Shopping list:

....

....

....

....

....

....

....

....

....

....

....

....

....

....

....

....

....

....

....

....

Your recipes
for the week

....

....

....

....

....

....

....

....

....

....

....

....

....

....

Eleventh week
Date: ....

List the things that make you feel good:

....
....
....
....
....

What you like about being pregnant:

1. ....

2. ....

3. ....

4. ....

5. ....

6. ....

7. ....

What you DON'T like about being pregnant:

1.

2.

3.

4.

5.

6.

7.

Your picture of the day

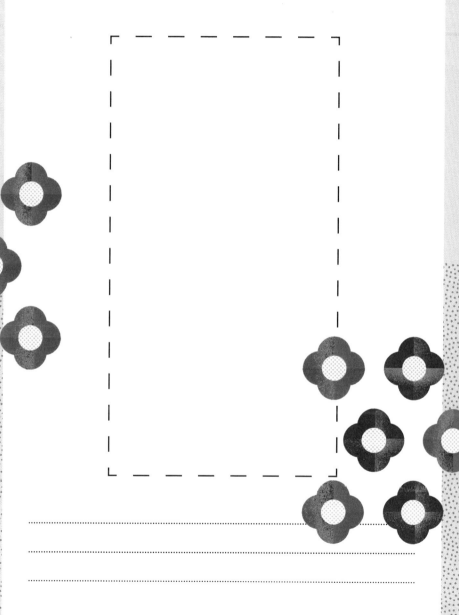

Twelfth week
Date: ....

Goals and challenges:

....
....
....
....
....

How often are you drinking water?

MONDAY

TUESDAY

WEDNESDAY

THURSDAY

FRIDAY

SATURDAY

SUNDAY

How often are you walking?

MONDAY

TUESDAY

WEDNESDAY

THURSDAY

FRIDAY

SATURDAY

SUNDAY

Books to read

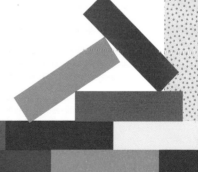

Now, What Can I Wear?

There are those who refuse to give up their style during pregnancy, those who are allergic to the phrase "maternity look," and those who think the only important thing is to be comfortable in any situation. Whichever team you feel you belong to, here are some tips for shopping in the coming months.

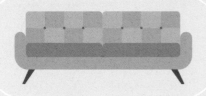

The Long-Live-Comfort Team

Finding comfortable (but cute!) maternity clothes is easy nowadays; most major brands have a line dedicated to mothers-to-be. If you prefer practicality, your favourite looks will definitely include loose pullovers or cardigans to leave unbuttoned, leggings and sneakers, along with loose-fitting dresses (especially in summer). These will keep you comfortable in any situation.

Another idea? Take a look in your partner's wardrobe for oversized T-shirts, shirts, jackets, or sweaters to get the most on a limited budget!

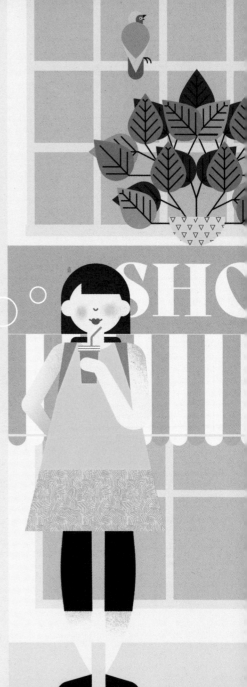

The Never-Give-Up-Style Team

Adopting a look that takes into account the transformations your body will go through during pregnancy does not mean you have to give up your style: just dial it back to the basics! One thing you must have in your wardrobe is at least one pair of maternity jeans that will allow you to combine style and comfort throughout your nine months. Shirts and T-shirts are best in a flowing, boyfriend-style. Another staple in the stylish mother-to-be's wardrobe is a pair of overalls in denim or some other soft fabric!

The Never-the-Maternity-Look Team

If the empire waistline really isn't your thing and your fashion icons are Rihanna and Ashley Graham, who even in pregnancy refused to give up their style, then have no fear: show off your new shape. Opt for close-fitting dresses and eye-catching accessories, and look for outfits that you can wear even after these nine months; for example, by buying a garment you like in a few sizes larger than usual. In any case, it is best not to neglect practicality: a soft shift or knit dress is better than a stretch shirt or suit, and a pair of leggings is more practical than low-rise jeans.

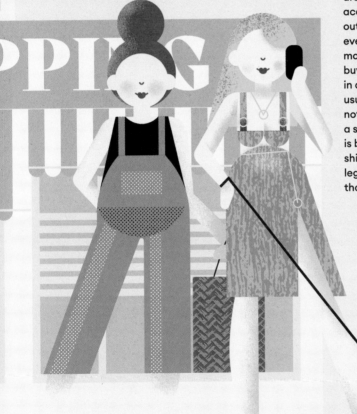

**Thirteenth week
Date:** ....

**List of clothes
to buy:**

1. ....
2. ....
3. ....
4. ....
5. ....

Things to do this week:

Unsolicited advice:

MONDAY

TUESDAY

WEDNESDAY

THURSDAY

FRIDAY

SATURDAY

SUNDAY

Who gives you energy now and why?

....

....

....

....

....

....

....

....

....

....

....

....

....

....

....

Fourteenth week

Date: ....

People who make you feel good:

....

....

....

....

....

Remember to:

....

....

....

....

....

....

....

....

....

....

Who makes you feel good?

People to avoid:

....

....

....

....

....

How you feel:

....

....

....

....

....

....

....

....

....

....

Make a list of all the things you are happy about

1. ....
2. ....
3. ....
4. ....
5. ....
6. ....
7. ....
8. ....
9. ....
10. ....
11. ....
12. ....
13. ....
14. ....
15. ....

Fifteenth week

Date: ....

Shopping list:

1. ....
2. ....
3. ....
4. ....
5. ....
6. ....
7. ....
8. ....
9. ....
10. ....
11. ....
12. ....

Words that describe you:

....
....
....
....
....
....

Words that DON'T describe you:

Attach
your sonogram
here

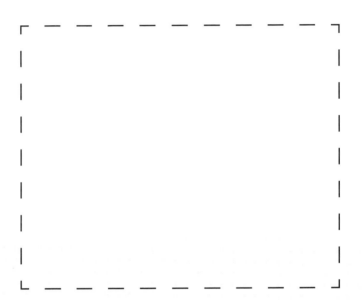

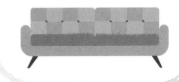

Sixteenth week
Date: ....

Goals and challenges:

....
....
....
....
....
....

....
....
....
....
....

How often are you drinking water?

How often are you walking?

MONDAY	MONDAY
TUESDAY	TUESDAY
WEDNESDAY	WEDNESDAY
THURSDAY	THURSDAY
FRIDAY	FRIDAY
SATURDAY	SATURDAY
SUNDAY	SUNDAY

Reflections about your sixteenth week of pregnancy

Hey, Can You Hear Me? The Development of a Baby's Senses

What does the baby perceive in the uterus? Can it hear our voices? What about smells? Every day, the foetus slowly grows and develops, and with it, its senses develop as well. At the seventh week of gestation, when it is the size of a grape, the foetus already develops its first sense, that of touch, and as early as the ninth week, it becomes a so-called "multi-receptive" being. Learn about the stages of development of the baby's senses in-utero!

Hearing and vision

Beginning in the eighth week, innervation of the inner ear begins and by the fifth month of gestation the baby's ears are already functioning! He or she will then be able to perceive voices, music and noises from the external environment, so well that loud ones may cause surprise or even fright! Relaxing music and speaking in soft tones are reassuring for your baby and are sounds that may be remembered even after birth. What about the baby's eyes? They may open in the seventh month of pregnancy, but sight is the last of the senses to develop because, in the darkness of the womb, there is little visual stimulation. The baby's vision will become more refined after birth.

Developing a sense of smell

Taste and smell develop hand in hand. From 11 weeks until birth, the taste buds located on the tongue become increasingly sensitive. In some way, what you eat will influence your child's tastes during his or her life!

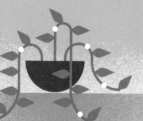

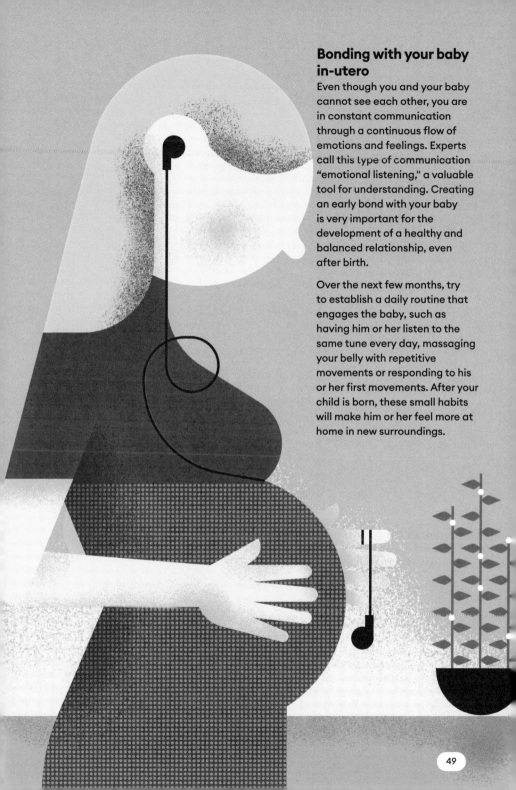

Bonding with your baby in-utero

Even though you and your baby cannot see each other, you are in constant communication through a continuous flow of emotions and feelings. Experts call this type of communication "emotional listening," a valuable tool for understanding. Creating an early bond with your baby is very important for the development of a healthy and balanced relationship, even after birth.

Over the next few months, try to establish a daily routine that engages the baby, such as having him or her listen to the same tune every day, massaging your belly with repetitive movements or responding to his or her first movements. After your child is born, these small habits will make him or her feel more at home in new surroundings.

Seventeenth week

Date: ....

Mum's playlist:

1. ....
2. ....
3. ....
4. ....
5. ....

6. ....
7. ....
8. ....
9. ....
10. ....

How you feel:

....

....

....

....

....

....

....

....

....

Visits and things to do:

MONDAY

TUESDAY

WEDNESDAY

THURSDAY

FRIDAY

SATURDAY

SUNDAY

Baby's playlist

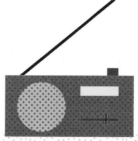

Eighteenth week

Date: ....

Recharge your batteries!

Things that energise you:

....

....

....

....

....

Things that tire you:

....

....

....

....

....

Other pregnant friends:

....

....

....

....

....

....

....

....

Appointments:

MONDAY ....

TUESDAY ....

WEDNESDAY ....

THURSDAY ....

FRIDAY ....

SATURDAY ....

SUNDAY ....

It's time to go out with your friends! What would you like to do?

Nineteenth week

Date: ....

Shopping list:

**What you would like
to do this week:**

....

....

....

....

....

....

**What you would
NOT like to do:**

....

....

....

....

....

....

Attach a picture of yourself here

....

....

....

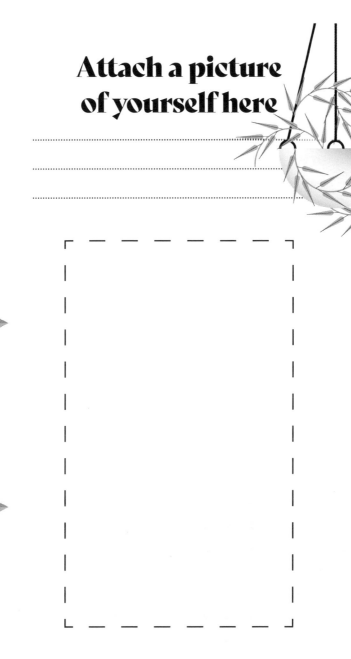

Twentieth week
Date: ....

New sensations as a mother:

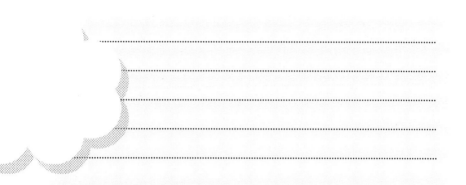

....

....

....

....

How often are you drinking water?

How often are you walking?

MONDAY	MONDAY
TUESDAY	TUESDAY
WEDNESDAY	WEDNESDAY
THURSDAY	THURSDAY
FRIDAY	FRIDAY
SATURDAY	SATURDAY
SUNDAY	SUNDAY

Think about what makes you feel good. Write it here:

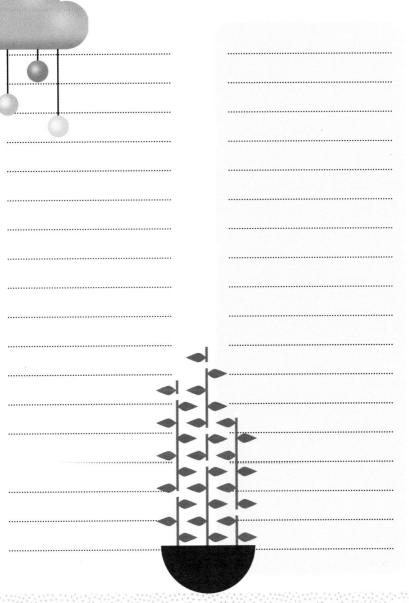

Twice the Joy, Twice the Love, Twice the Work: Having Twins

At the fifth- or sixth-week ultrasound, one out of eighty mothers discovers that she is expecting not just one baby, but two! As soon as the shock wears off, she will have a thousand questions, like what will my pregnancy be like? What about the delivery? What are the symptoms? What should I do? Here are some tips if you're having twins.

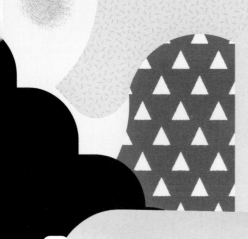

Types of twin pregnancies

Twin pregnancies can be divided into two groups:
- monozygotic: a single egg is fertilised by a single sperm and then splits into identical twins (one third of cases)
- dizygotic: two separate eggs are fertilised by two sperm, resulting in fraternal-twin siblings (two-thirds of cases).

Additional factors in determining the type of twin pregnancy are the number of placentas and amniotic sacs, which will be evident at the first- trimester ultrasound.

How many sonograms?

In bichorionic pregnancies (i.e., one placenta for each baby), one ultrasound scan per month is needed to follow the growth of the foetuses, the morphology and to evaluate any risk of premature delivery.

For the rarer monochorionic pregnancies (one placenta for two babies), get ready to have an ultrasound every two weeks in order to detect imbalances in the growth of the two foetuses.

In short, find a doctor you like to do your sonograms, because you will be seeing a lot of him or her!

Two babies, twice as tired

We are not all alike, and fatigue is very subjective, but it goes without saying that being pregnant with twins is more tiring than a "classic" pregnancy. Suffice it to say that having two babies often means suffering twice as much from nausea and that at six months, you already weigh as much as or more than a woman in her ninth month of pregnancy who is expecting a single baby.

Be careful to limit your sugar intake in order to avoid the risk of gestational diabetes and follow the advice of trusted midwives and gynaecologists to stay safe!

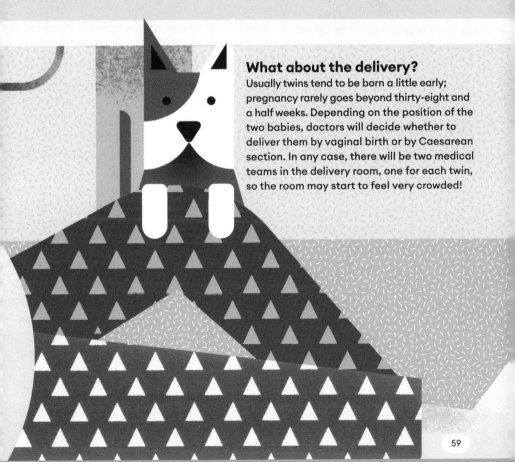

What about the delivery?

Usually twins tend to be born a little early; pregnancy rarely goes beyond thirty-eight and a half weeks. Depending on the position of the two babies, doctors will decide whether to deliver them by vaginal birth or by Caesarean section. In any case, there will be two medical teams in the delivery room, one for each twin, so the room may start to feel very crowded!

Twenty-first week
Date: ....

1. ....
2. ....
3. ....
4. ....
5. ....

Principal emotions of this week:

6. ....
7. ....
8. ....
9. ....
10. ....

People to see:

....
....
....
....
....
....
....
....
....
....

Visits and things to do:

MONDAY

TUESDAY

WEDNESDAY

THURSDAY

FRIDAY

SATURDAY

SUNDAY

Your recipes for the week

Twenty-second week

Date: ....

The reaction of others:

Questions you like:

Questions that annoy you:

....

....

....

....

....

....

....

....

Appointments:

Remember to:

MONDAY ....

TUESDAY ....

WEDNESDAY ....

THURSDAY ....

FRIDAY ....

....

....

....

....

....

....

....

SATURDAY ....

SUNDAY ....

What will your baby's personality be like? Make a list of what you expect

Twenty-third week

Date: ....

What you like about being pregnant:

....
....
....
....
....
....

What you DON'T like about being pregnant:

....
....
....
....
....
....

Shopping list:

....
....
....
....
....
....
....
....
....
....
....
....
....

Attach
a picture of yourself as a child

Twenty-fourth week

Date: ....

Goals and challenges:

....

....

....

....

....

How often are you drinking water?

How often are you walking?

MONDAY

MONDAY

TUESDAY

TUESDAY

WEDNESDAY

WEDNESDAY

THURSDAY

THURSDAY

FRIDAY

FRIDAY

SATURDAY

SATURDAY

SUNDAY

SUNDAY

Books on your bedside table, waiting to be read

....

....

....

....

....

....

....

....

....

....

....

....

....

....

....

....

From A to Z: Let's Think of a Name

Choosing a name should not be taken lightly: it is one of the elements that can characterise our personality. Some people choose their baby's name long before even having decided to have a child. For others, the process is a more difficult one, full of doubts and second thoughts. Is it better to choose an original name, or to stick to the classics? Should I trust the advice of friends and relatives, or ignore their preferences? Should I consider the etymology of the name, or only the way it sounds? Let's take a look at the various steps in choosing a name!

The character in a name

If you already have some ideas, consider the meanings of your ten favourites and of the names you think may have an impact on your baby's character. Try asking yourself what your child's personality will be like and what you consider the most important qualities in a person. Generosity? Fearlessness? The ability to listen or to be heard? Curiosity? Kindness? Candor? Based on your answers, think about the name that will best suit your child's character.

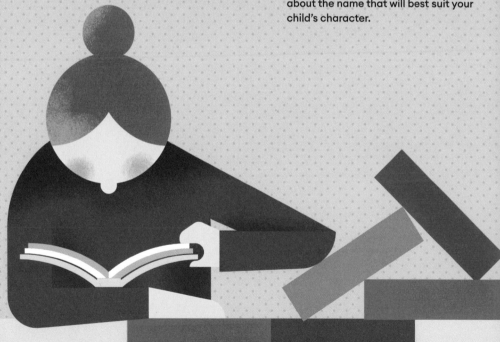

Surnames and traditions

The given name is always connected to one (or more) surnames. Try pronouncing the full name aloud. Does it sound right? If it is too difficult to pronounce or if you are not convinced, then consider other options. A word of advice: if the surnames are very long, choosing a short and simple first name is better. Some families have a tradition when it comes to choosing names. If that's not the case with yours, you can always draw inspiration from your (or your partner's) ancestors to come up with one that is interesting or meaningful. It might be a good way to honour someone who is no longer with you or to start a new tradition, such as choosing names with the same initials for all siblings.

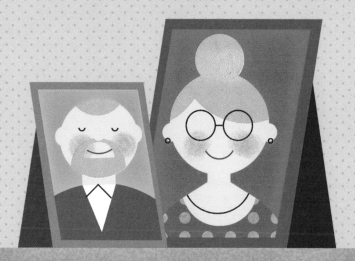

Looking for inspiration

To look for ideas that go beyond your family names, consider the names of the main characters in books you love, traditional names from your home town, the names of writers or artists you appreciate, as well as names in nature, astrology, mythology and history.

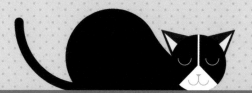

**Twenty-fifth
week
Date:** ....

Top ten names:

1. ....
2. ....
3. ....
4. ....
5. ....

6. ....
7. ....
8. ....
9. ....
10. ....

Visits and things to do:

How you feel:

MONDAY ....

TUESDAY ....

WEDNESDAY ....

THURSDAY ....

FRIDAY ....

SATURDAY ....

SUNDAY ....

....

....

....

....

....

....

....

....

....

....

Your recipes
for the week

Twenty-sixth week

Date: ....

Does the name define the person?

Names of pleasant people:

....

....

....

....

Names of unpleasant people:

....

....

....

....

How often the baby moves:

....

....

....

....

....

....

....

....

....

Remember to:

....

....

....

....

....

....

....

....

Do you have a recurring dream? Write it here if you do

Twenty-seventh week

Date: ....

Characteristics associated with your name:

....

....

People you've told about the name you've chosen:

....

....

....

....

....

....

....

....

....

....

....

....

....

....

....

....

People who don't like the name you've chosen:

....

....

....

....

....

....

....

....

....

....

....

....

Attach a picture
of yourself here

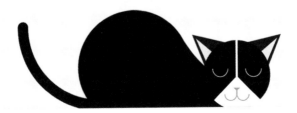

Twenty-eighth week

Date: ....

Goals and challenges:

....

....

....

....

....

How often are you drinking water?

How often are you walking?

MONDAY	MONDAY
TUESDAY	TUESDAY
WEDNESDAY	WEDNESDAY
THURSDAY	THURSDAY
FRIDAY	FRIDAY
SATURDAY	SATURDAY
SUNDAY	SUNDAY

The names of the main characters in your favourite books and movies

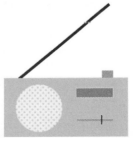

Good Night and Sweet Dreams

"Sleep tight!" is easier said than done when your belly gets bulky and your back starts to hurt. If you learn which positions are safest for the foetus (and most comfortable for you) along with a few other little tricks, you will actually be able to sleep tight again!

The best positions

The most recommended position is lying on your left side with your legs bent. This makes it easier for the blood to flow and carry oxygen to the foetus.

If you are used to sleeping on your stomach, for as long as the size of your belly allows you to, go ahead; you need not worry that the position will crush the baby, who is always protected by the amniotic fluid.

No hard-to-digest foods at dinner

Since many women suffer from digestive problems during pregnancy, it is best to avoid heavy and fatty dinners that may cause heartburn. If a little hunger pang strikes before bedtime, try eating some nuts, such as almonds or walnuts, that will give you a sense of fullness without weighing you down. If you suffer from acid reflux, opt for a position on your side with your head elevated.

Your new best friend: the pregnancy pillow

Pregnancy pillows are designed to facilitate lying on your side, to give you support and prevent back pain. There are many on the market, most of which belong to three types: "snake," "U-shaped," or "C-shaped." Usually you rest your head on the end of the pillow and hold the other between your knees. If you are a particularly light sleeper, opt for a pillow stuffed with polystyrene microbeads.

And know that your pillow will remain a faithful companion even after childbirth: it will be useful for breastfeeding.

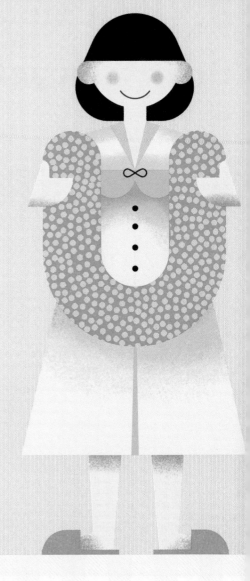

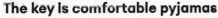

The key is comfortable pyjamas

During your pregnancy, your pyjamas should adapt to the changes in your body. Checking the comments left on various e-commerce sites, by other customers who have bought a pair you think you like, may be helpful.

The same is not true when it comes time to deliver. Hospitals usually ask that the mother-to-be wears a nightgown made from natural fibres that buttons down the front and a robe, rather than pyjamas.

Twenty-ninth week

Date: ....

For a good night's sleep:

1. ....
2. ....
3. ....
4. ....
5. ....

6. ....
7. ....
8. ....
9. ....
10. ....

Visits and things to do:

MONDAY

TUESDAY

WEDNESDAY

THURSDAY

FRIDAY

SATURDAY

SUNDAY

How you are sleeping:

....
....
....
....
....
....
....

Write down your thoughts about pregnancy

Thirtieth week
Date: ....

**What makes
you sleep well:**

Things that relax you:

....
....
....
....
....
....

Things that agitate you:

....
....
....
....

Appointments:

MONDAY ....

TUESDAY ....

WEDNESDAY ....

THURSDAY ....

FRIDAY ....

SATURDAY ....

SUNDAY ....

Unusual dreams
or nightmares

....
....
....
....
....
....
....
....
....
....
....
....
....
....
....
....

**Thirty-first
week
Date:** ....

**Top ten songs
to relax to:**

1. ....
2. ....
3. ....
4. ....
5. ....

6. ....
7. ....
8. ....
9. ....
10. ....

**Things you like
about being pregnant:**

....
....
....
....
....
....
....
....
....
....

**Things you DON'T like
about being pregnant:**

....
....
....
....
....
....
....
....

Attach a picture
of yourself here

Thirty-second week

Date: ....

Goals and challenges:

....

....

....

....

....

....

....

....

....

....

....

....

How often are you drinking water?

MONDAY

TUESDAY

WEDNESDAY

THURSDAY

FRIDAY

SATURDAY

SUNDAY

How often are you walking?

MONDAY

TUESDAY

WEDNESDAY

THURSDAY

FRIDAY

SATURDAY

SUNDAY

Movies to watch

1. ....
2. ....
3. ....
4. ....
5. ....
6. ....
7. ....
8. ....
9. ....
10. ....

Hypnobirthing & Relaxation

Have you ever heard of *hypnobirthing* or hypno-delivery? There is no hypnosis, swinging pendulums or drug use involved. Hypnobirthing is a form of meditation you can use to help manage your pain. It allows you to approach childbirth with serenity, while remaining present at all times so that you can enjoy the experience of your new child's birth fully. At the basis of this technique is a very simple assumption: the more you are afraid, the more pain you experience. And what are we afraid of? The unknown.

How to limit your fear and, with it, your pain

Human physiology plays a role in *hypnobirthing*. During childbirth, a woman produces oxytocin, a hormone responsible for uterine contractions and endorphins, which help to relieve pain and to relax. But when we are afraid, our bodies release adrenaline, which counteracts the beneficial effects of both oxytocin and endorphins! The result is stress that slows down labour.

The importance of mindfulness

Hypnobirthing puts mindfulness at the centre of the birth experience; it is the only way to truly relax. During labour, it is important to stay present and actively participate in the experience. If the mother-to-be makes independent, conscious decisions during labour, she is likely to be more serene in her relationship with the baby as well.

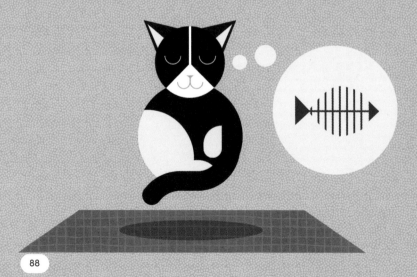

How is it possible to stay calm?

This is the time when you remember all the scenes in movies where doctors, friends and family are encouraging the mother-to-be to push as she gasps for breath and the tensions rise. Forget all of that! Focus intently on breathing, positive things you know about childbirth and relaxation techniques. We can be negatively conditioned by listening to the stories of other mothers who have experienced childbirth in a traumatic way. Instead, we should focus solely on our own experience and on positive thoughts. If we avoid concentrating on preconceived ideas, we can dispel the false tales that often accompany this moment.

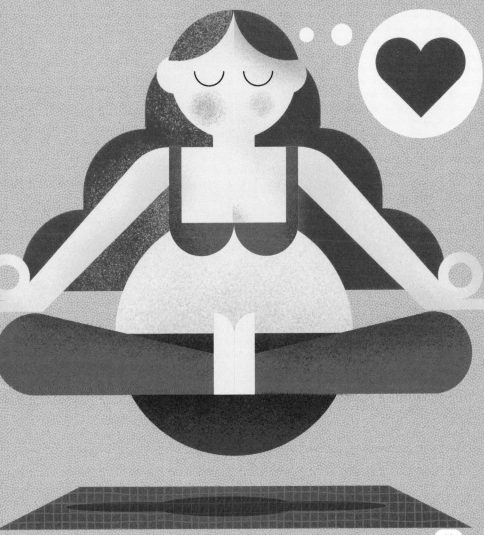

Thirty-third week

Date: ....

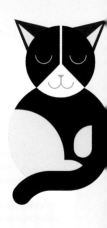

Your fears:

Visits and things to do:

How you feel:

MONDAY ....

TUESDAY ....

WEDNESDAY ....

THURSDAY ....

FRIDAY ....

SATURDAY ....

SUNDAY ....

Your motivational quotes

1. ....
....
....
....

2. ....
....
....
....

3. ....
....
....
....
....

4. ....
....
....
....
....

Thirty-fourth week

Date: ....

What makes you feel good?

Things that are good for me:

1. ....
2. ....
3. ....
4. ....
5. ....

Things I must avoid:

1. ....
2. ....
3. ....
4. ....
5. ....

Appointments:

Remember to:

MONDAY ....

TUESDAY ....

WEDNESDAY ....

THURSDAY ....

FRIDAY ....

SATURDAY ....

SUNDAY ....

Write down all the words that inspire well-being in you

Thirty-fifth week

Date: ....

Things that make you relax:

....

....

....

....

....

....

Shopping list:

Things that agitate you:

....

....

....

....

....

....

Attach a picture of yourself here

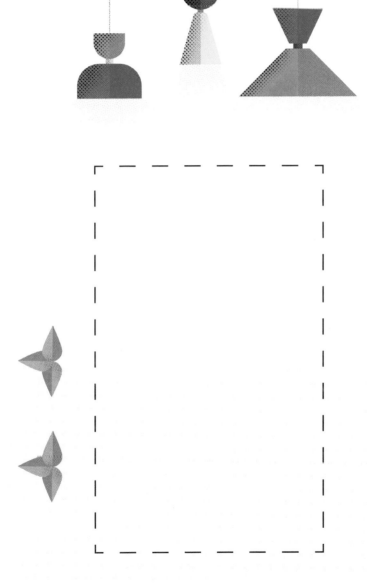

Thirty-sixth week

Date: ....

Goals and challenges:

....
....
....
....
....

How often are you drinking water?

MONDAY

TUESDAY

WEDNESDAY

THURSDAY

FRIDAY

SATURDAY

SUNDAY

How often are you walking?

MONDAY

TUESDAY

WEDNESDAY

THURSDAY

FRIDAY

SATURDAY

SUNDAY

What do you imagine delivery will be like?

Vaginal Birth or C-section? Delivery Is Always an Adventure!

Let's be clear: every pregnancy is different and no matter how much we anticipate what will happen, it may not go exactly as we planned. Having a birth plan and foreseeing how the baby will be delivered helps us prepare ourselves psychologically and dream a little; but we need to be ready to change course. Our thinking must be flexible and we should not get frustrated if things go differently from the way we imagined they would.

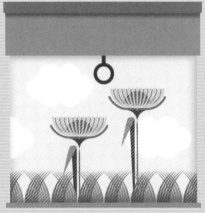

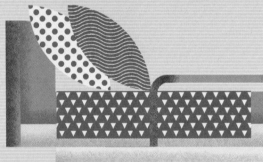

Vaginal birth

Vaginal childbirth, also called physiologic birth, can be the delivery of choice for a healthy mother whose pregnancy has been a smooth one and when the risk associated with delivery is low. You may choose to stimulate contractions using natural methods, but you may also choose to control pain with epidural analgesics administered under the supervision of a team of professionals (midwife, gynaecologist, anaesthesiologist and/or neonatologist).

The four phases of vaginal childbirth

Labour initiates with the prodromal phase, which is characterised by contractions and is followed by the dilation and expulsive phases. During the afterbirth phase, the placenta and membranes detach from the uterus and are expelled.

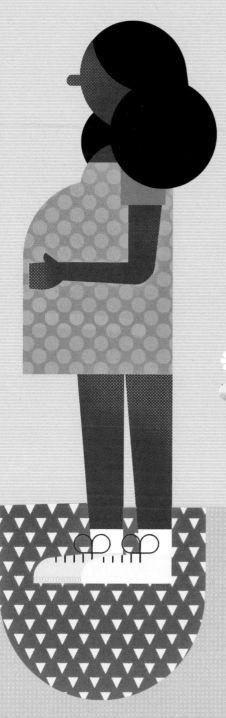

Positions during vaginal birth

The best position is definitely the one you choose. You are well aware of your body and have come to know its transformations during the course of your pregnancy.

That said, it is often the hospital where you decide to give birth that chooses the best position for you, based on the midwives' experience and assessment of your health. It is important to make your own choices, but it is just as important to trust and follow the advice of others and find a balance between the two. The most common positions are: lying down in the lithotomy position (introduced by Louis XIV, the Sun King); a squatting position; standing; on all fours; or in a lateral position.

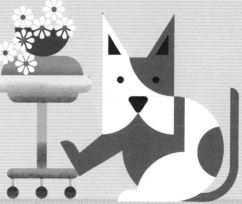

What about C-section delivery?

If for some reason the delivery looks like it is going to compromise the wellbeing of the mother or baby, a C-section is scheduled.

There are many false myths about this type of delivery that should be put to rest right away; the C-section scar will be almost imperceptible, given today's state-of-the-art surgical techniques; a C-section does not preclude the possibility of giving birth vaginally in future pregnancies; and a C-section has no negative effects on breastfeeding!

Thirty-seventh week

Date: ....

Final preparations:

1. ....

2. ....

3. ....

4. ....

5. ....

Visits and things to do:

How you feel:

MONDAY ....

TUESDAY ....

....

WEDNESDAY ....

THURSDAY ....

....

FRIDAY ....

....

SATURDAY ....

....

SUNDAY ....

What would you like to ask your doctor or midwife?

....
....
....
....
....
....
....
....
....
....
....
....
....
....
....
....
....

Thirty-eighth week

Date: ....

Things to remember:

What you will remember about being pregnant:

Things to forget:

Appointments:

MONDAY ....

TUESDAY ....

WEDNESDAY ....

THURSDAY ....

FRIDAY ....

SATURDAY ....

SUNDAY ....

Remember to:

....
....
....
....
....
....
....
....
....
....

Your expectations for the coming months

....

....

....

....

....

....

....

....

....

....

....

....

....

....

Thirty-ninth week

Date: ....

What you like about being pregnant:

1. ....
2. ....
3. ....
4. ....
5. ....
6. ....

What you DON'T like about being pregnant:

1. ....
2. ....
3. ....
4. ....
5. ....
6. ....

The first things to do as a new mother:

....
....
....
....
....
....
....
....
....
....
....
....
....
....
....
....
....

Attach a picture of yourself here

Fortieth week

Date: ....

Goals and challenges:

....
....
....
....
....

How often are you drinking water?

| MONDAY |
| TUESDAY |
| WEDNESDAY |
| THURSDAY |
| FRIDAY |
| SATURDAY |
| SUNDAY |

How often are you walking?

| MONDAY |
| TUESDAY |
| WEDNESDAY |
| THURSDAY |
| FRIDAY |
| SATURDAY |
| SUNDAY |

Your hopes

When the Wait Seems Never-Ending

Try not to get stressed over the continuous texts and phone calls from people wanting news about the baby. "So? Have you had the baby?", "Are we almost there?", "That baby wants to stay where it is." Stay calm. The expected date of delivery is an estimate: only four percent of babies are actually born on the expected day. Some are born before the due date, but most come after the forty-week deadline.

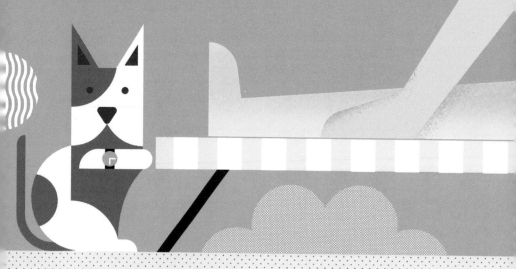

How long does pregnancy last?

On average, pregnancy lasts two hundred and eighty days, or forty weeks, from the first day of your last menstrual cycle. Birth before the thirty-seventh week of gestation is considered premature, birth between the thirty-seventh and forty-first weeks of pregnancy is full-term and birth at or after the forty-second week is considered post-term or protracted.

When is the decision to induce labour made?

If there has been no sign of contractions, the decision to induce labour is usually made between the 41st and 42nd weeks to avoid risk.

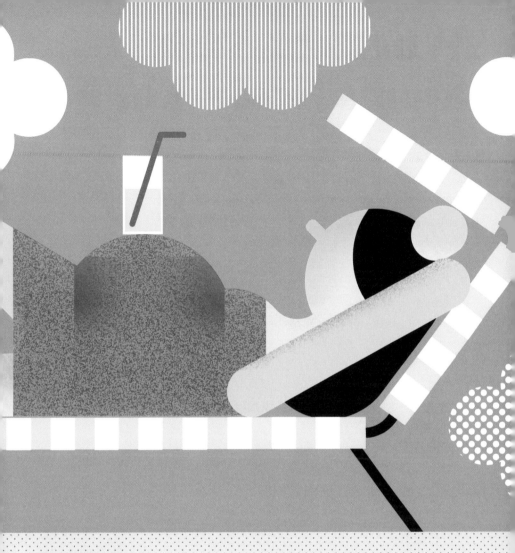

How can you induce labour?

After years of research, the answer is very simple: there is no way. Just relax and avoid looking at the calendar every two minutes.

It is often said that physical activity helps initiate labour, but it is not scientifically proven. Ideally, you should not disrupt your daily routine: walk if you feel like it, or take an afternoon nap if you prefer.

Only by being aware of your body and your feelings can you flow with the natural course of pregnancy. There are tips and tricks that may help unblock the situation, but they do not always work. Trust the doctors and midwives. They will do everything they can to avoid risks for you and your baby. They will guide you to the end of this adventure so that you can embark on the new and exciting one that is motherhood.

Forty-first week

Date: ....

What you will need after the baby is born:

1. ....
2. ....
3. ....
4. ....
5. ....

6. ....
7. ....
8. ....
9. ....
10. ....

Visits and things to do:

MONDAY ....

TUESDAY ....

WEDNESDAY ....

THURSDAY ....

FRIDAY ....

SATURDAY ....

SUNDAY ....

Impatience level:

MONDAY

TUESDAY

WEDNESDAY

THURSDAY

FRIDAY

SATURDAY

SUNDAY

Phrases that help you be patient

....

....

....

....

....

....

....

....

....

....

....

....

....

Forty-second week

Date: ....

Who do you want nearby?

Friends to call:

....
....
....
....
....

Friends to see:

....
....
....
....

Remember to:

....
....
....
....
....
....
....
....

Appointments:

MONDAY

TUESDAY

WEDNESDAY

THURSDAY

FRIDAY

SATURDAY

SUNDAY

Write down
all your good qualities,
push the negativity away

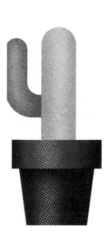

Attach your sonograms here

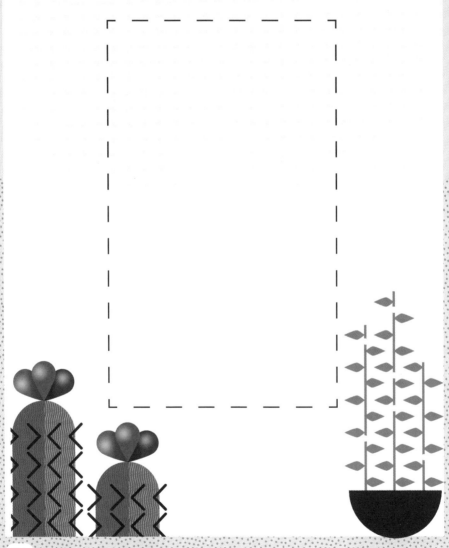

Attach your sonograms here

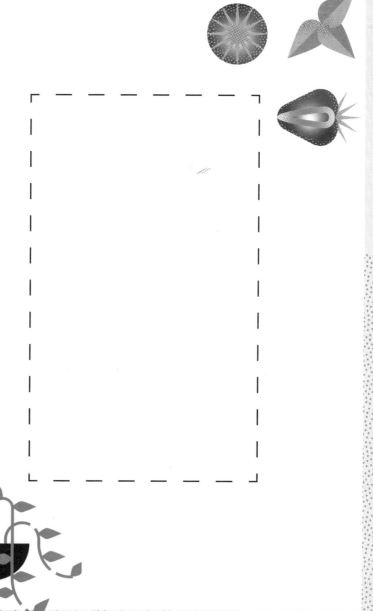

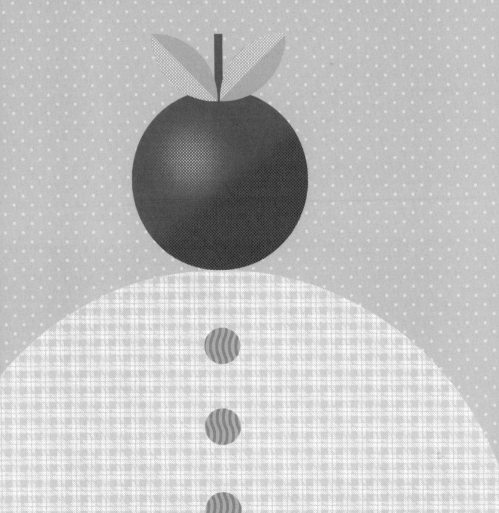

The Months

This adventure called pregnancy conventionally lasts 9 months. In medical circles, we prefer to speak of weeks of gestation. Dividing the pregnancy into months helps you to get oriented and organised and to live in the present more mindfully and serenely, without losing sight of the new life that awaits you.

In this section, you can record month-by-month the physical and psychological changes you are experiencing, the reactions of those around you, the results of the most important ultrasound scans and medical examinations and the hopes you have for the future that is now just around the corner!

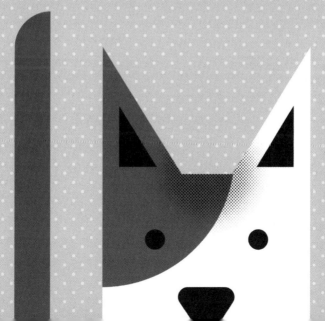

Pregnancy, You Make Me Tired!

Do you feel like you are not sleeping enough?

Do you keep waking up a thousand times, but right after the opening theme song of a movie, you fall sound asleep? Welcome to the first trimester!

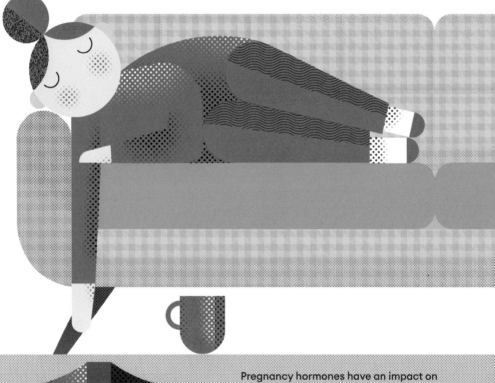

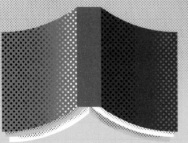

Pregnancy hormones have an impact on your body, your mood, your metabolism, your brain and even your sleep! Feeling tired all the time is completely normal in the first few months. Magically, your energy will be back in the second trimester. Take advantage of this energy to get ahead with your birth preparations, because when you get into the third trimester, fatigue will set in again.

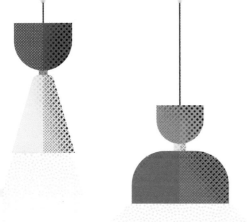

Let's bring back naps!

Don't feel guilty if you feel like you need a nap after lunch! It's a great way to catch up on some sleep after a night interrupted by bathroom visits to pee, restlessness and minor aches and pains. If your employer allows it, find a nice spot in the office to lie down and relax.

Count those sheep!

You need the right conditions to get a good night's sleep. Create a relaxing atmosphere and avoid too much screen time just before bed. Your room should be completely dark and the temperature should be slightly lower than the rest of the house.

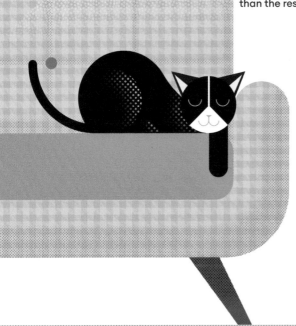

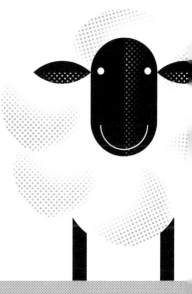

The amount of sleep you need undergoes dramatic changes during the course of your lifetime. An infant needs seventeen hours of sleep, but an adult may need even less than seven. What about you? A pregnant woman should sleep between eight and ten hours but, as always, it is subjective. If you feel rested after seven hours of sleep, there is no need to force yourself to sleep longer!

● Avoid caffeine, obviously. You can treat yourself to a cup of coffee after lunch but then, no more.
● Take care of yourself. What makes you feel good? A warm bath, a massage, reading a book on the couch, lighting a scented candle and listening to music. The things that give you serenity are the right things.

What movies do you find relaxing?

List five places where you can truly relax

And to Think You Were Just a Zygote!

The first trimester
The first trimester runs from conception to the twelfth week of gestation. Until the ninth week, the baby in your womb is referred to as an embryo; after the ninth week it is referred to as a foetus. By the twelfth week, all of its organs and limbs are formed, even if they are not yet functional. The foetus is about 6 cm (2.3 inches) long and weighs about 50 to 60 g (1.7 to 2.1 ounces).

The second trimester
The middle part of pregnancy, from the thirteenth to the twenty-eighth week, is considered the best, because the nausea and anxiety of the first months disappear. The baby's physiognomy is defined in this period and you can tell which sex your baby is.

Its heart works perfectly with accelerated beats of 110 to 160 per minute. At about twenty weeks, you can also begin to feel the baby move. At the twenty-eighth week, the foetus measures about 37 cm (14.5 inches) and weighs an average of 1,200 g (42 ounces).

The third trimester
Each week of this final stage of pregnancy, the foetus gains weight (nearly 200 grams per week) and is already beginning to look like a newborn.

Labour might begin at any time between thirty-seven and forty weeks. Gestation conventionally lasts forty weeks, but it is not uncommon for it to last as long as forty-one weeks and five days (to learn more go to "When the Wait Seems Never-Ending" section).

At birth, babies are measured according to the Apgar index to evaluate their appearance and overall health. Average weight is 3,300 g (116 ounces) and average length is 45–50 cm (17 to 19 inches).

Twenty-four hours after conception, the first cell formed by the meeting of the two gametes, the zygote, begins to grow into an embryo and then into a far more complex organism called a foetus. This growth process will last about forty weeks, until the time of delivery. What are the stages of prenatal development?

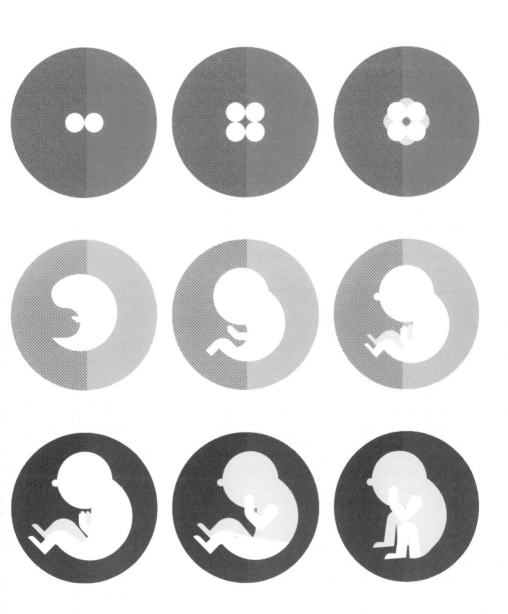

Start daydreaming: What do you expect from these nine months?

....
....
....
....
....
....
....
....
....
....
....
....
....
....

What are you feeling right now? What your life is like today

I Have News for You. . . .

Fun ways to announce your pregnancy

Is there anything more exciting than sharing good news with the people you love? If you've been dying to shout it to the whole world ever since you found out you were pregnant, these are some fun ways to do it.

For future dads and future grandparents, for your other children and friends, make the announcement a moment to remember.

How to tell your friends

● Invite your closest friends to dinner and when it is time for dessert, instead of the usual cake, bring jars of baby food to the table!
● You can use social media to inform friends that are far away. Take a photo of each family member's shoes and add a pair of baby shoes to the lineup.
● Take a photo of two large breakfast cups with a baby bottle in the centre: simple and memorable.

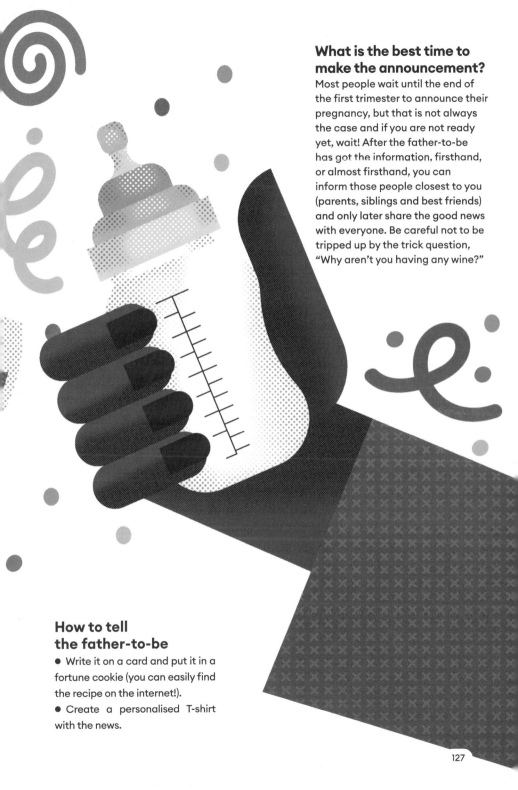

What is the best time to make the announcement?

Most people wait until the end of the first trimester to announce their pregnancy, but that is not always the case and if you are not ready yet, wait! After the father-to-be has got the information, firsthand, or almost firsthand, you can inform those people closest to you (parents, siblings and best friends) and only later share the good news with everyone. Be careful not to be tripped up by the trick question, "Why aren't you having any wine?"

How to tell the father-to-be

● Write it on a card and put it in a fortune cookie (you can easily find the recipe on the internet!).

● Create a personalised T-shirt with the news.

What about your announcement? How did you share the news to your friends and family?

....
....
....
....
....
....
....
....
....
....
....
....
....
....
....
....

What was a positive or negative reaction that surprised you most?

The Magical Second Trimester!

With the fourth month, the period considered the sweetest and happiest of pregnancy begins—the magical second trimester. No more of the nausea and anxieties you experienced in the first months. This is the time to develop a real (albeit symbiotic for now) relationship between you and your baby.

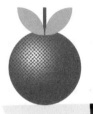

Here is a partial (not necessarily universal) list of the changes taking place in your body:

- Your belly is rounder (your uterus grows about 4 centimetres per month).
- Your centre of gravity changes as the pelvis prepares for the baby to pass through it.
- A dark line called the "linea nigra" may appear between your pelvic region and your navel.
- Your breasts grow larger and your weight increases.
- Your hair becomes stronger and shinier thanks to hormones.
- You may experience ligament pain.
- You may need to step into the bathroom to pee more often than usual.

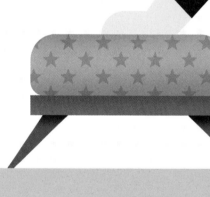

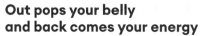

Out pops your belly and back comes your energy

By now your belly no longer goes unnoticed and you feel like telling everyone, literally everyone, that they are seeing right: you're pregnant and now you can say so!

This is the moment that you will reach a state of harmony and emotional stability that is difficult to put into words. The exhaustion of the first trimester is water under the bridge: now you are full of energy, but be careful not to overdo it. Listen to your body and go at nature's pace.

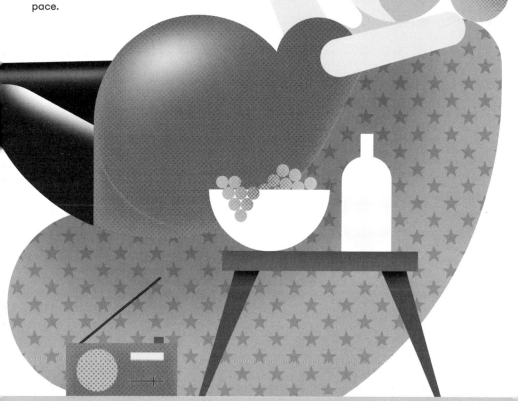

That first little kick

Beginning at 18 weeks, you will be able to feel your baby's first movements, an event that will confirm symbiosis between you. Foetal movements and the presence of a new life that is growing become tangible and it will be easier to interact with your baby, who at this point will begin to recognise your voice.

Your first times as a mother:

....
....
....
....
....
....
....
....

....
....
....
....
....
....
....
....

Your body is changing. What do you like about the new you?

Your Newborn's Room: Mission Creativity

The saying goes, "those who have time wait for no time." This applies to preparing your newborn's room, too.

Now that your hormones are your friend and your energy is back, it's time to shop, before your belly grows more and fatigue sets in again. What are you waiting for?

It is time to launch into one of the most fun and creative pregnancy projects. Here are our tips for preparing a complete list.

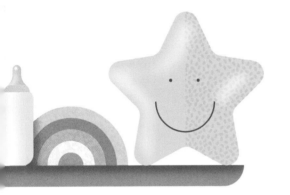
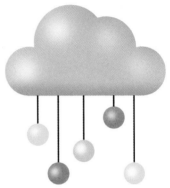

The essentials . . .

- Crib or bassinet: your newborn is used to the protected and familiar environment of prenatal life and may feel lost in a bed that is too big. For the first few months, therefore, a bassinet is preferable; but if you choose to buy a crib right away, just add a crib reducer and some soft fabric bumper rails.
- Changing table: since you'll never be able to leave your newborn alone on the changing table, you'll need a table with several compartments to keep wipes and diapers readily available. Make sure the surface is washable, obviously.
- Closet with shelves or chest of drawers to store your baby linens (baby blankets and sheets need some room) and baby clothes. Having what your baby uses most at your fingertips is fundamental.
- Choose soft colours for the nursery walls such as grey, white, beige, or dusty pink. Soft, muted wall colours will favour your baby's restfulness.
- Breastfeeding chair: to make breast or bottle-feeding more enjoyable, you need to be comfortable, to be able to rest your back and perhaps rock.
- Lights: to make the atmosphere warm and welcoming, choose soft lights, for example a table lamp or floor lamp.

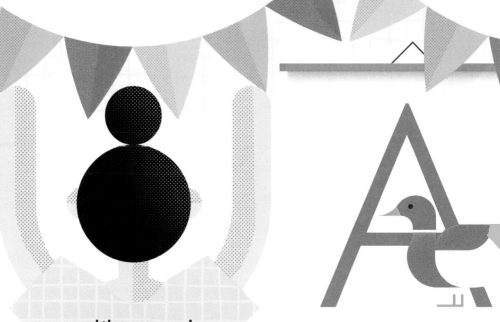

. . . and the accessories

- Decorative wall stickers.
- Small shelves for books
  and knick-knacks
  or a Montessori-style
  bookcase.
- Large baskets
  for stuffed animals.
- Colourful garlands with flags,
  pompoms or lights.
- Paintings and drawings
- Colourful carpet
  or soft puzzle carpet.
- Infant jungle gym.

ABCDEFGHIKLMN
OPQRSTUVXYZ

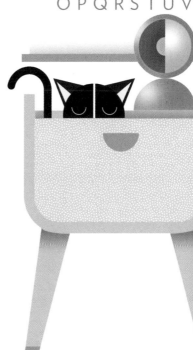

Furniture, decorations and lights to buy:

1. ....

2. ....

3. ....

4. ....

5. ....

6. ....

7. ....

8. ....

9. ....

10. ....

Which books will be in your baby's first library?

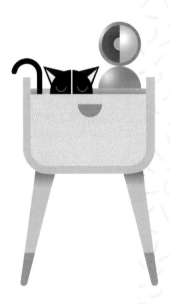

Your Birth Plan

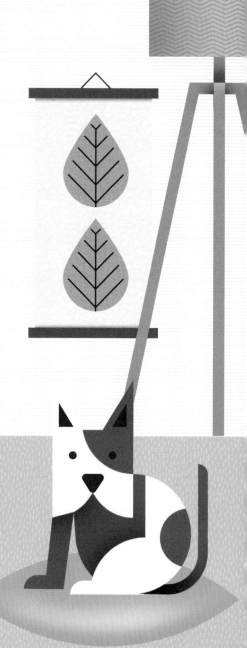

Pregnancy is an exciting, adventurous journey, but it is also difficult to predict with certainty because it may be full of unexpected events and surprises. Drawing up a birth plan and defining your preferences with respect to childbirth with the people involved (from your partner to the midwife) will help you clear up your doubts and feel more at ease. Drawing up your plan is something we can help you with!

What is a birth plan and why is it useful?

A birth plan is simply a list of your wishes with respect to the time of your labour and delivery, the hospital environment in which you would like to find yourself and the medical attention you would like to receive for yourself and your newborn. Sharing your plan with your gynaecologist and midwife could provide them with some important pointers on how to make this moment more harmonious.

In short, in drawing up a plan, you will make a useful checklist for managing the next steps of your pregnancy, which is useful, especially if you are someone who likes being in control or at least feeling like you are. But remember, If you don't feel the need to make a plan, simply let go and approach this wonderful experience with flexibility and an open mind.

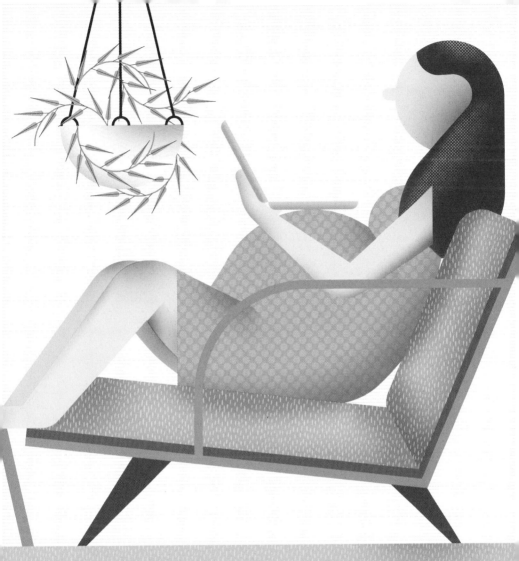

An example of a birth plan

Try answering these questions about your needs and wants. Ignore the ones that you feel are unimportant:

- If the hospital allows it, who would you want beside you during labour?
- If the hospital allows it, would you like the labour to be accompanied by special music?
- During labour, would you prefer to walk around, lie down, take a shower or bath, sit on a ball, be massaged, etc.?
- Would you like to request epidural anaesthesia?
- In case of vaginal childbirth, in what position would you like to give birth?
- Would you like the umbilical cord to be cut by a particular person of your choice?
- Do you think you would like to donate the blood from the umbilical cord?

Write your answers, together with your partner

How many examinations have you done so far?

Get Your Suitcase Ready!

It is always advisable to avoid any unnecessary anxiety! The best thing to do is to get ready and get it over with. Get out your travel bag or a small suitcase and we'll help you pack what you need! After giving birth, depending on whether the delivery was vaginal or a C-section and on whether the mother or child have special needs, the hospital stay is usually two or three days. Pack clothes for the entire stay, which includes labour, delivery and the baby's first days.

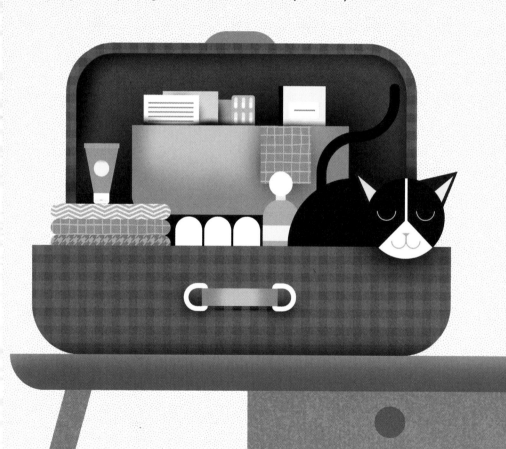

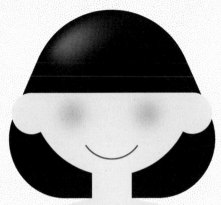
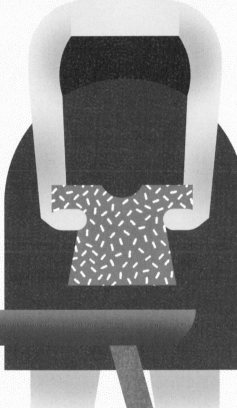

The indispensable

First of all, remember to pack the documents that you may need, such as medical records, sonograms and personal identification and insurance cards.

And then, something comfortable for the delivery:

- a nightgown for childbirth
- a robe
- a sweater or sweatshirt
- a jumpsuit
- pyjamas (or leggings and T-shirt, whichever you prefer)
- lots of underwear
- large cotton pads
- towels
- shampoo and shower gel
- shower slippers
- bedroom slippers
- nursing bra

And for your newborn?

- 6/8 bodysuits
- 6/8 one or two-piece PJs
- 3/4 pairs of socks
- cotton and/or chenille onesies
- bibs
- hats
- wool or cotton blanket or, even better, a sleep sack
- baby soap

Details are important

In addition to the essentials, do not underestimate the importance of the things that may be considered superfluous but that are fundamental for your well-being, such as music and podcasts, massage oil, books and something delectable to munch on.

143

Now it's your turn! Free rein in making your own list:

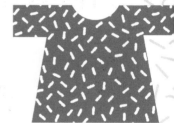

1.

2.

3.

4.

5.

6.

7.

8.

9.

10.

Do you follow any influencer mums? Who are your favourites?

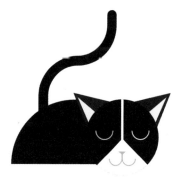

When the Nest is Ready

In the third trimester, you need to start preparing for the new life that is coming, not just your baby's, but your own as well. This is a time when you may have mixed, conflicting emotions. On one hand, you can't wait to hold your child in your arms; and on the other, you wish the symbiotic harmony that binds you together would never end. But don't worry: as usual, your hormones will take care of it! At this stage of pregnancy, oxytocin steps in. Let's learn more about it!

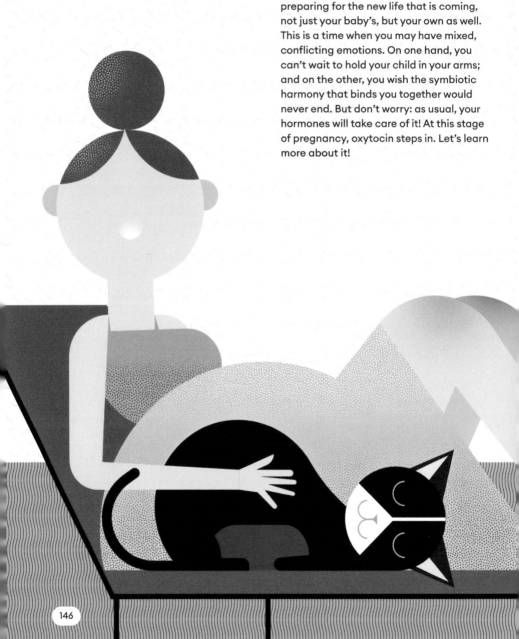

What does oxytocin do?

It is no coincidence that oxytocin is known as the "love hormone." At this stage of pregnancy, it helps you create an emotional bond with your baby, acting on the brain as a neurotransmitter. It decreases levels of anxiety and aggressiveness and encourages empathy and the so-called nesting instinct—the desire to prepare everything you need to welcome your newborn, just like other animals do.

During labour, oxytocin is responsible for initiating your uterine contractions so, if for some reason its production is interrupted, it may be administered in the form of a pharmaceutical.

But when is the journey over?

Beginning in the eighth month, you may experience feelings of impatience, of heaviness and of fatigue. This journey of pregnancy is beautiful, but you may start to want to arrive at your destination. During this period, it is not uncommon to go from "I can't wait to meet my baby" to "Help! Who will this stranger be?" If you are experiencing mixed emotions, just accept them. They are part of the journey and probably will not end at delivery, but will continue into the first months of your newborn's life and of yours, as a mother.

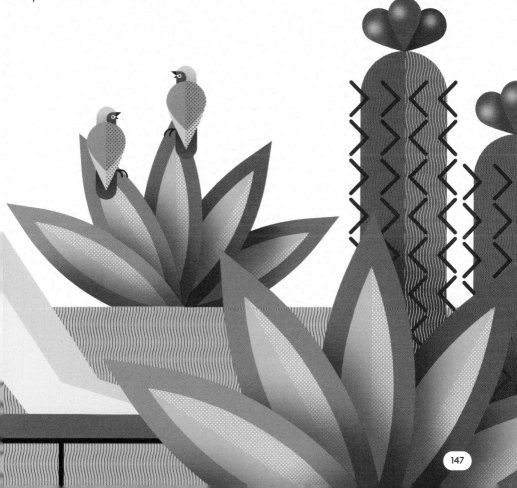

How do you feel?
Let your pen
describe your emotions:

....
....
....
....
....
....
....
....
....
....
....
....
....
....

Dedicate some time to your favourite activities: which ones?

Next Stop: A New Life

At 36 weeks, putting on your socks has probably become an impossible feat, which is quite normal since you are in your ninth month now. At this point, you should have gained from 9 to 12 kg (but this is an average; it could be more or less). If you gave birth now, your baby would no longer be considered premature, but normally, contractions begin at 38 weeks. Let's see what happens with mother and with baby!

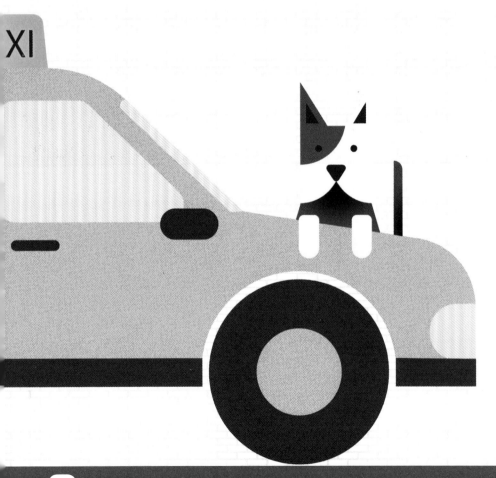

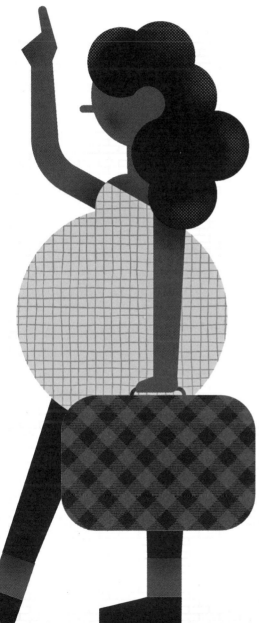

The mother

You have chosen a name; the baby's room and other essentials are ready; your suitcase for the hospital is as well; you have completed the prenatal course; if your employer allows it, you have already started your maternity leave — what else is there to do? Well, nothing, except to wait. For many mothers-to-be, this last period can be tiring, especially physically. Doctors and midwives recommend resting as much as possible during this month. As your baby's weight increases, you too will feel heavier, a feeling exacerbated by the fluid retention that is typical of this phase. You will feel the first preparatory contractions and the spike in hormones may cause mood swings and restlessness.

The baby

Inside your belly, your baby is also preparing to come into the world. The respiratory system is working well, ready to take its first breath of air and the digestive system is also ready. In this final month, the foetus's biggest job is to gain weight (you'll feel it because it will start pushing more and more on your pelvis and lower abdomen). What are the signs of the onset of labour? When contractions become more intense and closer together (5 or 6 per hour) it means you are approaching the big moment. Your water breaking is another clear sign that you are almost there and it is time to go to the hospital. When in doubt, it is best to make a phone call to your midwife or maternity ward. Who is going with you to the hospital? Now is the time to think about it. Your amazing adventure with the little creature inside you is far from over and will continue to evolve. Enjoy every milestone and welcome to your new life!

To-do list: rest, complete final preparations and remember to bring your prenatal exams

1. ....

2. ....

3. ....

4. ....

5. ....

6. ....

7. ....

8. ....

9. ....

10. ....

Useful phone numbers and names of people to contact before delivery

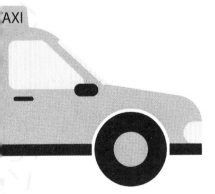

There Are Nine, but They Fly By!

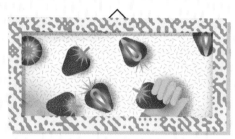

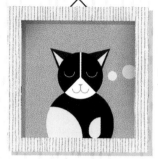

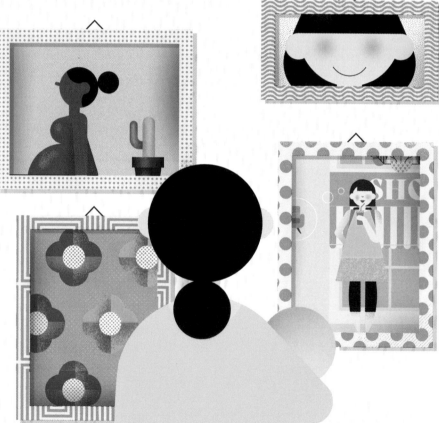

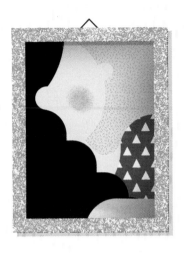

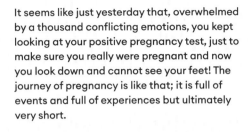

It seems like just yesterday that, overwhelmed by a thousand conflicting emotions, you kept looking at your positive pregnancy test, just to make sure you really were pregnant and now you look down and cannot see your feet! The journey of pregnancy is like that; it is full of events and full of experiences but ultimately very short.

Are you one of those curious readers who immediately skips to the last part of the book first, instead of diligently reading about the progression of the weeks and months? If so, no spoilers! Start from the beginning and I'll see you back here later!

During these nine months, you will be building your family's future. For that, you need to take a look at the path you have travelled.

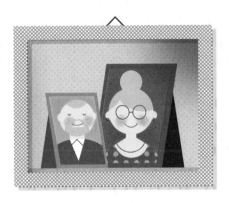

Look back at the past but prepare for the future

A few years from now, you will be able to turn the pages of this journal together with your son or daughter and everything will feel different. These months are a unique opportunity to think about the future you would like for yourself and your family, to lay the foundation for a new life. If you have recorded not just things to do and appointments, but also your feelings and emotions in the pages of this journal, you have created a precious document; one that clearly explains who you have been, who you are now and who you will be to anyone who reads it.

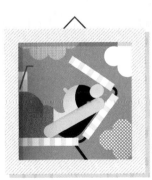

In order to lay the foundation for your future, you need to look back to your past, to your childhood and, even earlier, to your parents and grandparents, all the way back to your ancestors. Try tracing your roots by creating a family tree, together with those closest to you, of the ancestors who brought you here today, expecting a child of your own.

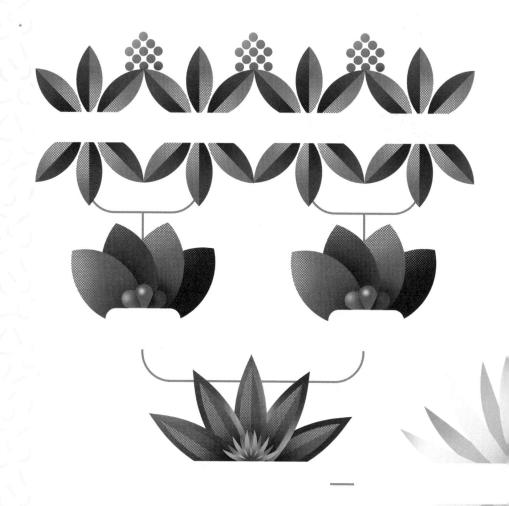

Family tree

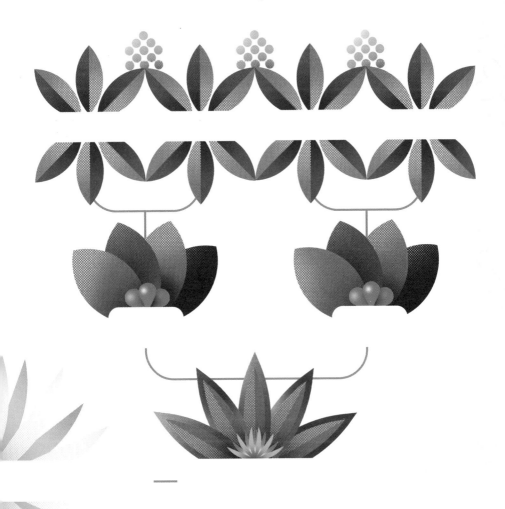

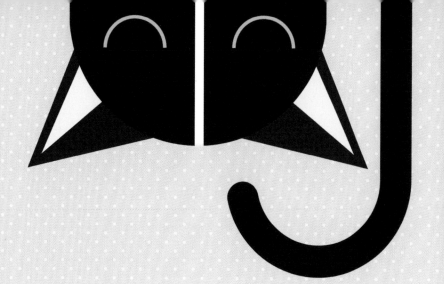

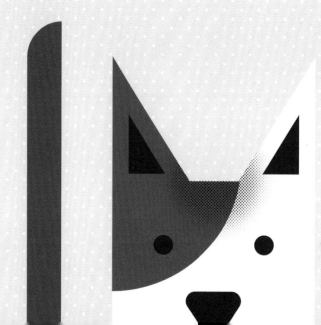

Lara Pollero lives and works between Milan and Savona, Italy. After graduating with a degree in Philosophy, she followed her passion for art and publishing, which soon became her profession. After working as an editor for the contemporary art magazines *Flash Art* and *Kaleidoscope*, she began collabourating with major Italian publishing houses and then moved to Paris, where she began translating miscellaneous and non-fiction books by night while working as a web content editor for a French company specialising in online media production during the day. Today she continues to enthusiastically pursue various publishing projects, while wondering how she also manages to be a mum of twins.

Alice Iuri is an Italian illustrator. After studying Philosophy and Industrial Design in Venice, she started working as a graphic designer until she joined *The*World*of*DOT studio in Milan in 2016. Meanwhile, she continued to explore and experiment in the world of illustration, focusing mainly on portraits, where she merges her technical training with her humanistic education. Her illustrations have been published by numerous publishing houses and magazines, including *Linus* and *Internazionale,* as well as being included in prestigious group exhibitions. She has a dog, which often appears on her Instagram page: @alice_iuri_illustrator.